Rim Khemakhem
Rahma Gargouri

Pain in palliative care: evaluative and therapeutic approaches

Rim Khemakhem
Rahma Gargouri

Pain in palliative care: evaluative and therapeutic approaches

ScienciaScripts

Cover image: www.ingimage.com

This book is a translation from the original published under ISBN 978-620-6-70781-3.

Publisher:
Sciencia Scripts
is a trademark of
Dodo Books Indian Ocean Ltd. and OmniScriptum S.R.L publishing group

120 High Road, East Finchley, London, N2 9ED, United Kingdom
Str. Armeneasca 28/1, office 1, Chisinau MD-2012, Republic of Moldova, Europe
Printed at: see last page
ISBN: 978-620-7-35922-6

PLAN

INTRODUCTION

The incidence of cancer in the world continues to rise, with ten million people affected in 2000 according to the WHO, and as many people expected to be affected by 2020(1). Advances in treatment have turned a large number of cancers into chronic diseases. Seventy percent of cancer sufferers will experience pain during their illness. This pain needs to be managed, sometimes on a long-term basis.

Around 80% of patients with cancer present one or more painful sites. Of these, 30% have severe pain(2, 3).

Defined by the IASP (International Association Against Pain), pain is "an unpleasant sensory and emotional experience associated with actual or potential tissue damage, or described in terms of such damage"(4).

Pain is an important symptom for which patients seek relief. As a result, a well-managed analgesic treatment must enable the patient and those around him to maintain a quality relationship throughout the course of the disease. Controlling cancer pain is therefore a priority in oncology, requiring multidisciplinary assessment and management.

In this study, we set out to assess cancer pain control and the prevalence of anxiety and depressive disorders in the course of bronchopulmonary cancer (PBC), as well as their correlation with pain.

PATIENTS AND METHODS

We performed a cross-sectional study in the Thoracic Oncology Unit of the Pneumology Department of the HédiChaker University Hospital of Sfax between March and August 2018 in patients with confirmed PBC.

1. INCLUSION CRITERIA

Patients with confirmed PBC who are regularly monitored in the Pneumology Department of the CHU HédiChaker.

2. DATA COLLECTION

The following data were collected from the patients' medical records: age, sex, co-morbidities, socio-economic status, histological type, stage of disease, metastatic sites and average consultation time.

Pain was assessed before and after analgesic treatment, differently according to its type, by :

- Visual Analogue Scale (VAS): this scale consists of a horizontal line ranging from "no pain" to "maximum unimaginable pain". The patient indicates the level of pain on the line by positioning a cursor. The pain score is displayed on the other side of the scale (Figure 1).

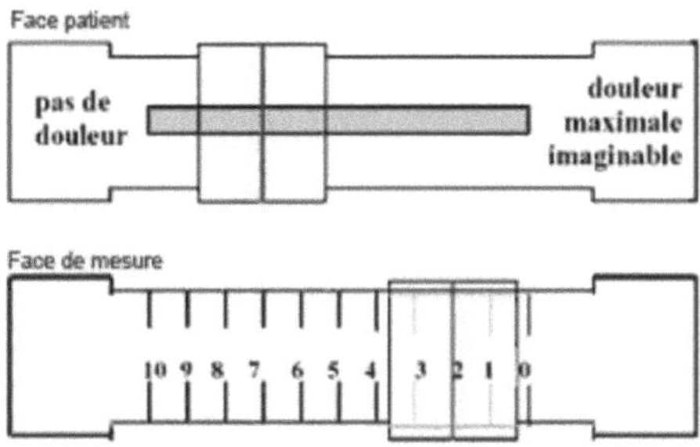

Figure 1: Visual analogue scale

• The DN4 Questionnaire (5): The DN4 questionnaire is a screening tool for neuropathic pain. It comprises seven items for questioning the patient and three for clinical examination of the patient. These items are grouped into 4 questions. For each item, the patient answers "yes" or "no".

At the end of the questionnaire, each "yes" is counted. If the patient's score is equal to or greater than 4/10, the test is positive (Figure 2).

QUESTION 1 : la douleur présente-t-elle une ou plusieurs des caractéristiques suivantes ?

	Oui	Non
1. Brûlure	☐	☐
2. Sensation de froid douloureux	☐	☐
3. Décharges électriques	☐	☐

QUESTION 2 : la douleur est-elle associée dans la même région à un ou plusieurs des symptômes suivants ?

	Oui	Non
4. Fourmillements	☐	☐
5. Picotements	☐	☐
6. Engourdissements	☐	☐
7. Démangeaisons	☐	☐

QUESTION 3 : la douleur est-elle localisée dans un territoire où l'examen met en évidence :

	Oui	Non
8. Hypoesthésie au tact	☐	☐
9. Hypoesthésie à la piqûre	☐	☐

QUESTION 4 : la douleur est-elle provoquée ou augmentée par :

	Oui	Non
10. Le frottement	☐	☐

OUI = 1 point NON = 0 point **Score du Patient : /10**

Figure 2: DN4 questionnaire

In addition, the patients included answered questionnaires relating to anxiety-depression using the Hospital Anxiety Depression (HAD) test(6) with its Arabic version. Also known as the "emotional repercussion scale". It is used to assess the patient's emotional and affective state. The patient reads the questionnaire and underlines the answer that best expresses this state.they feel. A score was assigned to each response. Psychological distress was considered when the score was > 10.

3. STATISTICAL ANALYSIS :

The statistical study was carried out using SPSS 20 software. Qualitative variables were compared using the Chi 2 test and quantitative variables using the Student test. The statistical significance threshold was set at 5%. In the comparative study of qualitative variables, the Chi 2 test was used; if the sample was small, the Fischer (P) test was used. We studied the correlation between two quantitative variables using Pearson's r correlation test.

RESULTS

1- Epidemiological characteristics

1.1. Age and gender :

The study included 77 patients, 99% of whom were male. The mean age was 64.87 ± 9.14 years, with extremes ranging from 43 to 88 years. Half the subjects (50.6%) were over 65 (Figure 3).

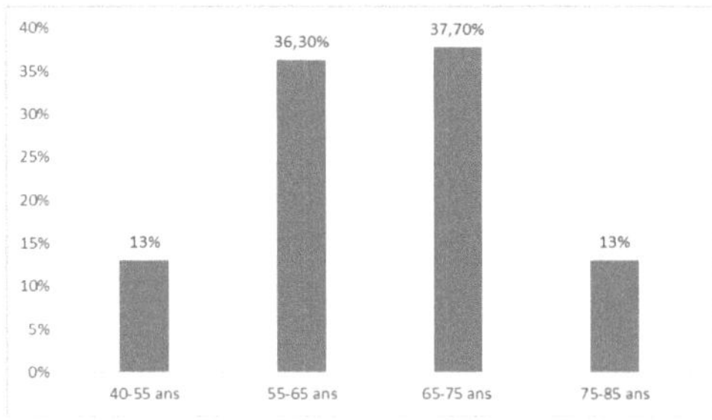

Figure 3: Distribution of subjects by age.

1.2. Level socio-economic

Socioeconomic status was average in 63% of patients and low in 36% of cases (Figure 4).

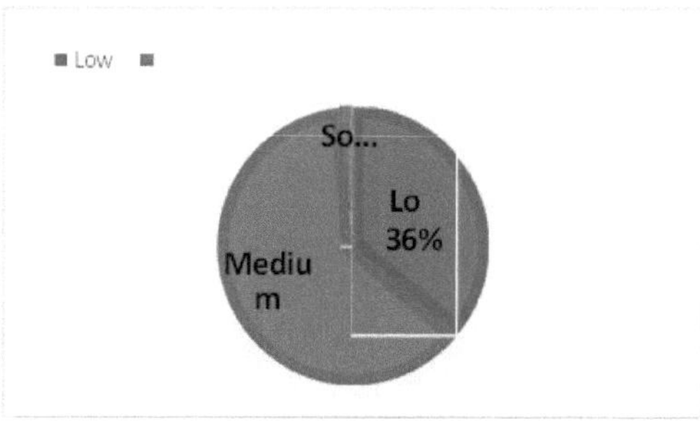

Figure 4: Patients' socio-economic levels

1.3. Medical history

A pathological history was present in 17% of patients. These were mainly cardiovascular co-morbidities (arterial hypertension, rhythm disorders, diabetes).

2- Characteristics of pathology tumours

The average consultation time was 176.7 ± 146 days. The most common histological type was non-small cell carcinoma (85.7%). The latest TNM classification was used for staging the disease, with the tumour classified as stage IV in 69.7% of cases, IIIB in 25.8%, IIIC in 3% and IIIA in 1.5% (Figure 5).

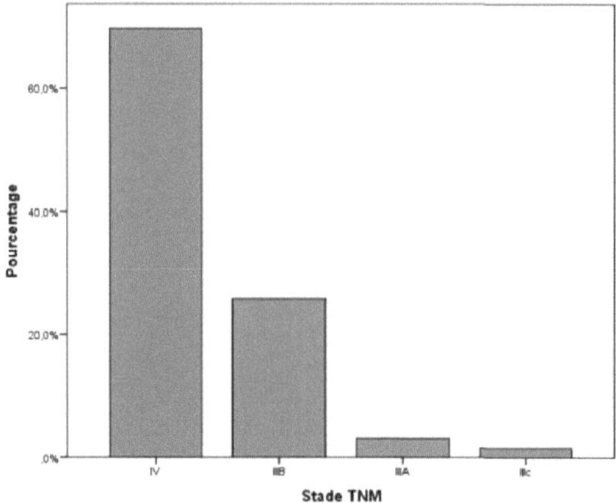

Figure 5: Tumour classification according to the 2017 TNM classification Metastases were present in 69.7% of cases.

Poly metastases were present in 18.8% of patients. Cerebral metastases were the most frequent (15.5% of cases) (Table I).

Table I: Main metastatic locations

Location	Percentage
brain	15,5%
Lung	14,1%
bone	9,6%
adrenal	3,1%
hepatic	1,6%

3- Assessment of the psychological state of patients

According to the HAD score, 26% of patients suffered from anxiety and 25% from depression (Figure 5).

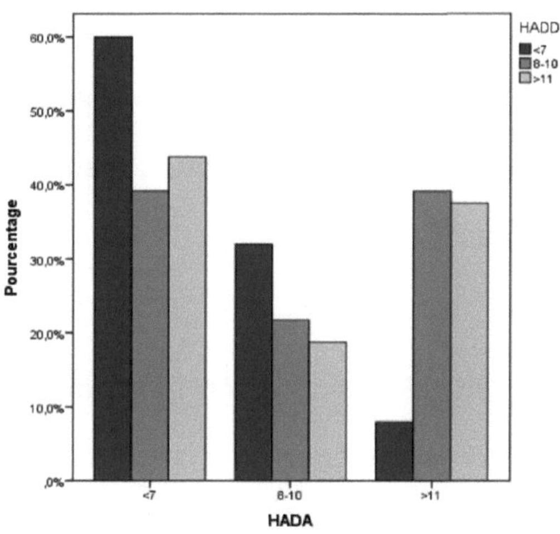

Figure 5: Patients' anxiety-depressive states

HADA: HAD anxiety score

HADD: HAD depression score

No significant correlation was found between anxiety and depressive disorders and age, socio-economic level, disease progression, tumour stage or metastatic site.

4- Pain assessment and treatment

- Pain assessment before treatment

Pain was nociceptive in 92.1% of cases and mixed in 7.9%. The mean VAS score before treatment was 5.17 ± 3.07. Fifty-five per cent of patients had a VAS score greater than or equal to 5. Thirty-six percent of patients had a VAS score of less than 3, 25% between 3 and 7 and 39% greater than or equal to 7.

- Treatment

Approximately 28% (28.4%) of patients used morphine-type tier III analgesics, with an average daily dose of 62.94 ± 42.97 mg (Figure 6).

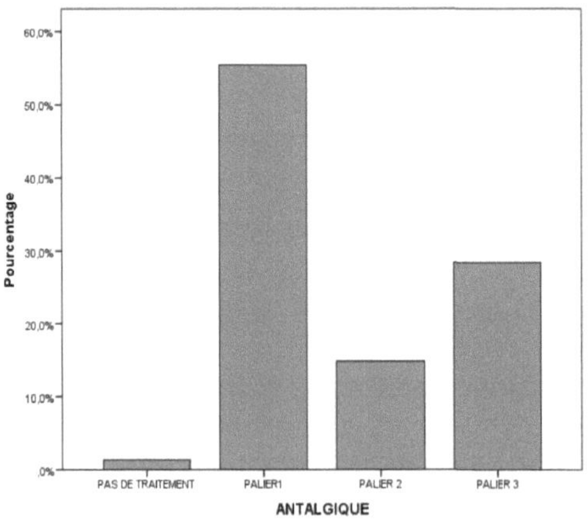

Figure 6: Use of analgesics for pain control

•Pain assessment after treatment

The mean VAS score after treatment was 2.53 ± 2.41 under treatment (on the day of inclusion). Eighteen percent of patients had a VAS score greater than or equal to equal to 5. Seventy-one percent of patients had a VAS score of less than 3, 22% between 3 and 7 and 7% greater than or equal to 7.

•A significant correlation was found between depression (p=0.042), pain intensity before treatment (r=0.60; p=0.00) and the level of pain control. Indeed, it seems that the presence of a depressive disorder increases the intensity of the pain experienced by the patient. Thus, the existence of a depressive disorder has a negative effect on pain control (Figure 7).

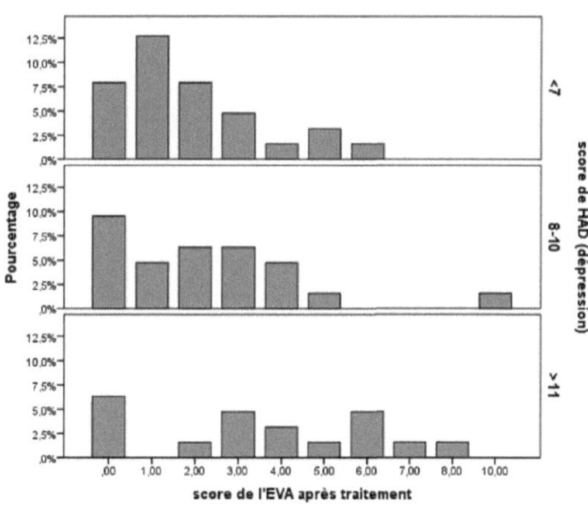

Figure 7: VAS score according to patients' psychological profile

- However, no correlation was found between age ($r=0.15$; $p=0.18$), anxiety ($p=0.5$), tumour stage ($p=0.53$), metastatic site ($p=0.33$) and lack of pain control.

DISCUSSION

The control of cancer pain is a very important objective, both in outpatient care and in health establishments. Advances in treatment have turned a large number of cancers into chronic diseases. In fact, most people with cancer will suffer from pain throughout their illness, requiring treatment, sometimes over the long term.

1- Assessment of pain

The WHO defines pain assessment as "the first vital step in the management of cancer pain". It also sets out a number of recommendations for its implementation (7). Poor pain assessment is one of the main barriers to good patient management. Pain assessment is therefore essential and must be carried out systematically before any treatment is introduced and throughout the course of treatment.

1-1- Objectives

Pain assessment enables an appropriate therapeutic strategy to be put in place. Nociceptive pain, resulting from tissue damage, is not treated in the same way as neuropathic pain, linked to damage to the nervous system. Nociceptive pain can be acute or chronic. All these types of pain can also vary in intensity: from mild to unbearable. There are also so-called psychogenic pains, which have no lesion-related origin and certainly linked to the patient's psychological state. These different types of pain require different treatments. It is therefore important to characterise them as precisely as possible in order to implement appropriate treatment (7-9). Cancer-related pain occupies a special place because it can present all these characteristics, sometimes at the same time. Pain assessment helps to identify patients in pain, because not all patients express their pain, and just because a patient doesn't complain doesn't mean he or she isn't suffering. It also facilitates communication between patient and carers. The use of pain assessment methods also means that the results can be kept in the patient's care file. This makes it easier to decide on the therapeutic strategy to adopt, and enables better monitoring of the effectiveness of the treatment. This assessment must take place in hospital and at each outpatient consultation.

1-2- Relations with patients

The relationship with the patient is not always easy. They can sometimes be frustrated or resigned to their pain, and in some cases even aggressive. To avoid this, you need to show empathy and be available and willing to listen(10). Some patients express their pain spontaneously, while others hide it for various reasons. It is therefore important to establish a relationship of trust with the patient. Any pain expressed must be taken into account, even if there is no obvious lesion. Because pain is a subjective phenomenon, it is the patient who is best placed to talk about it. You also need to be able to explain that the causes of pain are often multifactorial and complex.

1-3- When should pain be assessed ?

Pain must be assessed both at the start and throughout the course of treatment and each time new elements appear (11). This imperative seems is well established in the practice of the majority of responding doctors and should be encouraged. However, a small proportion of doctors do not assess pain, or do so only when the patient complains. The WHO considers pain assessment to be "the vital first step in the management of cancer pain"(7), so it is likely that the management of these patients could be improved. In a medical thesis evaluating the management of cancer pain by GPs in Paris, 90.9% of the doctors questioned assessed pain at each consultation, while 4.3% never assessed it. In another study, evaluating the management of cancer pain by GPs in Rennes, they found that 89% of GPs assessed pain at each consultation(12).

1-4- At

A proper assessment of pain in patients with or without cancer begins with a somatic assessment, i.e. an aetiological work-up. Pain assessment must also include an assessment of the patient's psychosocial context(9, 10).

•Somatic assessment

This assessment should be carried out at the time of the initial complaint, whenever there is a change in the pain symptomatology, and whenever new signs appear (Table II). The aim is to define the pathophysiological mechanisms(13).

Table II: Details of the clinical description of pain

Description of pain	
Circumstances of onset	Seniority of the pain Mode of onset. Concurrent life events, Initial diagnosis
Description of the pain	topography, type of sensation intensity, Aggravating or relieving factors
Evolving profile	Permanent, recurring, intermittent...
Previous and current treatments	Medicinal or non-medicinal Doses, duration and methods of administration Beneficial and undesirable effects
Impact	Anxiety, disorder of sleep, disabilities, functional or professional
History and pathologies	Associated personal, family, evolving history, If

Psychosocial assessment

Psychosocial assessment concerns all patients suffering from chronic pain, whether cancerous or not. It can be carried out in collaboration with a specialist doctor (psychiatrist or psychologist). To achieve this, it will be necessary to obtain the support of the patient, who may see this approach as a refusal by the doctor to recognise his or her pain. On the contrary, the patient should see the psychiatrist as a specialist in certain drugs or analgesic techniques (psychotropic drugs, hypnosis, etc.) and as a fully-fledged player in the assessment of chronic pain (8-10, 13, 14). Depression is common in persistent painful conditions. According to an American study, among 405 cancer patients, 68% of whom were suffering from pain (15), almost half had depression associated with her pain. It seems that the combination of depression and pain has an amplifying effect on each other. (16). According to a study published in 2004, depression is two to three times more common in cancer patients than in the general population(17), which is similar to the results found in our study. Depression can lead to resistance to certain therapies and modify pain behaviour. A personality disorder often leads to pain becoming established (18). However, in our study, no correlation was found between anxiety and lack of pain control. It should also be noted that most patients are unaware of the nature and stage of their illnesses. This can influence the patient's psychological state, reducing anxiety and reinforcing feelings of depression, which are linked to the functional symptoms of the disease, such as fatigue, anorexia, impairment of general condition and their impact on quality of life. The important thing is to allow the patient to formulate his thoughts and interpretations. The aim is to better understand, clarify and correct the misunderstandings of these pain sufferers. In this way, the patient can adopt a more appropriate approach to their pain.Patients sometimes use their complaints (verbal or gestural) to communicate with those around them. This is known as the "relational dimension" of pain (9, 10, 13). There are scales for assessing functional disability, although these are more commonly used in rheumatology (EIFEL, Dallas, SF36 and the ANAES chronic pain impact scale)(19, 20).

2- Pain management

There are generally three types of pain, depending on the pathophysiological processes involved. Nociceptive pain, neuropathic or neurogenic pain and psychogenic pain. These different types of pain often coexist. This is known as mixed pain.

- **Nociceptive pain**

Nociceptive pain is treated with analgesics of the three WHO(7) levels .at doses adapted to their intensity. Morphine is a typical example in oncology. WHO recommendations on the management of cancer pain are based on five main principles(7, 21) :

- The first concerns the oral route. This should be preferred wherever possible. In the event of contraindication (dysphagia, gastrointestinal obstruction, vomiting, etc.), the rectal or subcutaneous route may be used.

- Treatment should be given at regular intervals and the next dose should be administered before the effect of the previous dose has worn off. This ensures continuous relief. Interdoses (or rescue doses, boluses) are provided in the event of acute pain peaks. An interdose can contain 50 to 100% of the dose administered over 4 hours. Titration should be carried out systematically at the start of treatment or whenever treatment changes, to determine the appropriate doses.

- the degree of intensity of the treatment must respect the three levels

of analgesia.

1) Non-opioid analgesics for mild to moderate pain (EV<3).

2) weak opioids for moderate to severe pain (3<EVA<7).

3) strong opioids for intense to very intense pain (VAS>7).

The transition from one level of analgesic to another is made in sequence, if the pain is not relieved or is of increasing intensity. For each level, it is possible to use a co-antalgesic to increase the efficacy of the initial analgesic or reduce its dosage. Level 1+2 and 1+3 combinations are possible, but two opioid drugs cannot be administered simultaneously.A strong opioid can be used directly if the pain is very severe. intense. In its 2012 recommendations, the European Association of Palliative Care (EAPC) even suggests treating certain mild to moderate cancer pain with strong opioids, with dosage adjustments (11);

- prescriptions are personalised:

Unlike tier 1 or 2 analgesics, strong opioids do not have clearly defined usual or maximum doses. They are adapted to each patient after titration, and the dose used is that which provides pain relief and is well tolerated.

- prescriptions must be optimised. Administrations should be regular and adapted to the patient's lifestyle. The time of going to bed and getting up should be taken into account, and doses should be spread throughout the day.

The aim is to achieve constant pain relief and optimum management of undesirable effects. This involves rigorous monitoring, with traceability of doses and times of administration of analgesics. In our series, pain was nociceptive in 92.1% of cases. Approximately 28% of patients were using level III analgesics of the morphine with a mean daily dose of 62.94 ± 42.97 mg. The mean VAS score before treatment was 5.17 ± 3.07 and 2.53 ± 2.41 under treatment.

• **Neuropathic pain**

Cancer neuropathic pain has characteristic properties that distinguish it from nociceptive pain. This type of pain affects between 19% and 39% of cancer patients suffering from pain (22). They may be of variable origin:

✓ Peripheral (paraneoplastic neuropathy) ;

✓ inducedby an anticancer (taxanes, salt of thalidomide, vincristine);

✓ inflammatory ;

✓ by tumour compression, tumour plexopathy, etc.);

✓ central (spinal cord injury due to tumour compression, thalamic or brainstem tumour injury).

This pain is poorly relieved by conventional analgesics of the WHO levels. This is because there is no tissue lesion stimulating the nociceptors. The aim will therefore be to prevent spontaneous nociceptive discharges and to combat a defective nociceptive nervous system. Two classes of drugs are used as first-line treatments: antidepressants (tricyclics and SNRIs) and anti-epileptics. Only certain molecules are concerned and have marketing authorisation for the treatment of neuropathic pain. However, these treatments, which have only been validated for short periods and whose benefit/risk ratio must be assessed on a case-by-case basis, have generally only shown partial efficacy. It is therefore important to define realistic objectives with patients, so that their pain can be described as "acceptable".In our series, 7.9% of patients had nociceptive pain, 7% of whom were treated with pregabalin.

•Psychogenic pain

Psychogenic pain, on the other hand, is difficult to define and is highly subjective. It is thought to be due to a lowering of the pain perception threshold and to psycho-affective disorders.

3- Pain that refuses treatment

Rebellious cancer pain is pain for which specific treatments do not bring about any improvement, or pain that causes excessive adverse effects that are not controlled by symptomatic treatments. There is no real consensus regarding their management. However, the French National Agency for the Safety of Medicines and Health Products published recommendations for good practice in 2010 on the subject of intractable pain in advanced palliative situations in adults(23). These concern the off-label use of certain drugs. These include

- ✓ Perimedullary, parenteral and topical local anaesthetics;
- ✓ fentanyl and sufentanil ;
- ✓ ketamine ;
- ✓ MEOPA ;
- ✓ methadone ;
- ✓ midazolam ;
- ✓ morphine via the perimedullary and intracerebroventricular routes;
- ✓ propofol.

Stubborn cancer pain can also be treated by interventional

therapies, such as radiology for small tumours (liver, lung, kidney, etc.) or cementoplasty for bone metastases. In 2013, the French Society of Anaesthesia and Intensive Care (SFAR) and the French Society for the Study and Treatment of Pain (SFETD) also published recommendations on locoregional analgesic techniques for cancer pain (24). There are therefore a number of therapeutic strategies and exceptional routes of administration used in advanced palliative situations. In our series, no patient benefited from one of these strategies.

4- Pain control cancer

Managing cancer pain can be difficult for many doctors. This is consistent with most of the literature on the subject(12). The difficulties most frequently reported concern the treatment itself. According to them, it can be complicated to find an effective treatment, at effective doses, while achieving a suitable level of tolerance and as few adverse effects as possible. This notion is regularly expressed in the literature(25, 26).

Doctors then cite the management of drug interactions, the issue of addiction to treatments (morphine in particular) and problems of patient compliance, which may be partly the result of the preceding notions. Difficulty in assessing pain (lack of time, characterisation of pain) was found by almost 30% of doctors. Pain assessment is time-consuming and the time available for consultation is often limited (27). This is followed by the management of intractable cancer pain and the psychological component of pain, as well as the fear of treatment (mainly morphine, associated with the end of life). The 2002 study published in the journal "Douleurs", concerning pain management, emphasised that the main difficulties encountered by doctors in managing patients were compliance, tolerance of analgesics and pain assessment. Doctors also cited the dosage and efficacy of analgesics, self-medication, the psychological aspect of pain, time management in consultations, dosing schedules and drug interactions(28). These issues could probably be addressed through therapeutic patient education programmes.

CONCLUSION

The incidence of new cases of cancer in France has risen sharply over the last thirty years. More than half of cancer patients suffer from pain. Pain is often difficult to treat because of its different components and its progressive nature. Treating pain is a priority. In this perspective, we conducted a cross-sectional study carried out in the Thoracic Oncology Unit of the Pneumology Department of the Hédi Chaker University Hospital of Sfax between March and August 2018 in patients with confirmed PBC. According to the type of pain, it was assessed by the visual analogue scale (VAS) before and after treatment and by the DN4 Questionnaire for neuropathic pain. In addition, the patients included completed questionnaires relating to anxiety-depression (ADH). Psychological distress was considered to exist when the ADH was > 10. The study included 77 patients. The mean age was 64.87 ± 9.14 years. The mean time to consultation was 176.7 ± 146 days. The most common histological type was non-small cell carcinoma (85.7%). The tumour was classified as stage IV in 69.7% of cases. Pain was nociceptive in 92.1% of cases. The mean VAS score before treatment was 5.17 ± 3.07 and 2.53 ± 2.41 under treatment (on the day of inclusion). Approximately 28% (28.4%) of patients were taking morphine-type tier III analgesics, with a mean daily dose of 62.94 ± 42.97 mg. Twenty-six percent of patients suffered from anxiety and 25% from depression. A significant correlation was found between depression (p=0.042), pain intensity before treatment (r=0.60; p=0.00) and pain control. On the other hand, no correlation was found between age (r=0.15; p=0.18), anxiety (p=0.5), tumour stage (p=0.53), metastatic site (p=0.33) and non-control of pain. Despite its frequency, pain is often inadequately treated in patients with primary bronchopulmonary cancer. For optimal management of these patients, repeated and close reassessment of their pain is essential. We also need to screen for and treat anxiety and depressive disorders in patients, most of whom are in stage IV, where quality of life is paramount. The results show that the main difficulties encountered by doctors lie in correctly assessing certain types of pain, implementing a treatment that is sufficiently effective yet well tolerated, monitoring patients between consultations and managing the psychological component of pain.

APPENDICES

Appendix 1: Visual analogue scale

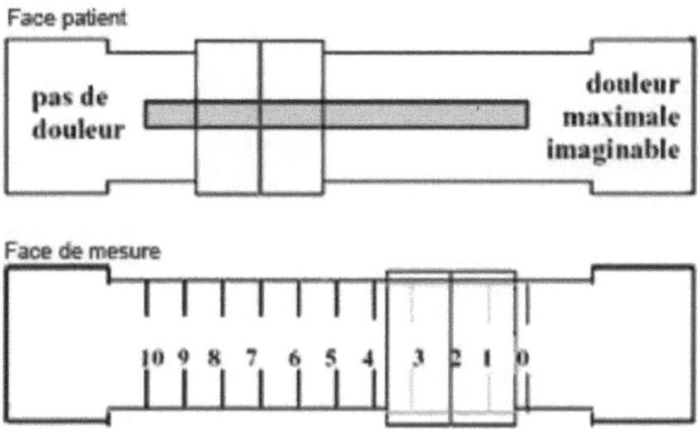

According to the setd-douleur.org website

Appendix 2: DN4 questionnaire

QUESTION 1 : la douleur présente-t-elle une ou plusieurs des caractéristiques suivantes ?

	Oui	Non
1. Brûlure	☐	☐
2. Sensation de froid douloureux	☐	☐
3. Décharges électriques	☐	☐

QUESTION 2 : la douleur est-elle associée dans la même région à un ou plusieurs des symptômes suivants ?

	Oui	Non
4. Fourmillements	☐	☐
5. Picotements	☐	☐
6. Engourdissements	☐	☐
7. Démangeaisons	☐	☐

QUESTION 3 : la douleur est-elle localisée dans un territoire où l'examen met en évidence :

	Oui	Non
8. Hypoesthésie au tact	☐	☐
9. Hypoesthésie à la piqûre	☐	☐

QUESTION 4 : la douleur est-elle provoquée ou augmentée par :

	Oui	Non
10. Le frottement	☐	☐

OUI = 1 point **NON = 0 point** **Score du Patient : /10**

According to the institut-upsa-douleur.org website

Appendix 3: TNM classification 8th EDITION

T - Tumeur	Tx	Tumeur primaire non connue ou tumeur prouvée par la présence de cellules malignes dans les sécrétions broncho-pulmonaires mais non visible aux examens radiologiques et endoscopiques.
	T0	Absence de tumeur identifiable.
	Tis	Carcinome *in situ*.
	T1	Tumeur de 3 cm **ou moins** dans ses plus grandes dimensions, entourée par du poumon ou de la plèvre viscérale, sans évidence d'invasion plus proximale que les bronches lobaires à la bronchoscopie (c'est-à-dire pas dans les bronches souches).
	T1a(mi)	Adénocarcinome minimalement-invasif
	T1a	≤ 1cm
	T1b	> 1 cm et ≤ 2 cm
	T1c	> 2 cm et ≤ 3 cm
	T2	Tumeur de **plus de 3 cm, mais de 5 cm ou moins**, avec quelconque des éléments suivants : -envahissement d'une bronche souche quelle que soit sa distance par rapport à la carène mais sans envahissement de la carène, -envahissement de la plèvre viscérale, -existence d'une atélectasie ou pneumonie obstructive s'étendant à la région hilaire ((sub)lobaire ou pulmonaire)
	T2a	> 3 cm mais ≤ 4 cm
	T2b	> 4 cm mais ≤ 5 cm
	T3	Tumeur de **plus de 5 cm et de 7 cm ou moins**, ou associée à un(des) **nodule(s) tumoral(aux) distinct(s) et dans le même lobe**, ou ayant au moins l'un des caractères invasifs suivants : -atteinte de la paroi thoracique (incluant les tumeurs du sommet), -atteinte du nerf phrénique, -atteinte de la plèvre pariétale ou du péricarde.
	T4	Tumeur de **plus de 7 cm** ou associée à un(des) nodule(s) pulmonaire(s) distinct(s) comportant un envahissement quelconque parmi les suivants : -médiastin, -cœur ou gros vaisseaux, -trachée, -diaphragme, -nerf récurrent, -œsophage, -corps vertébraux, -carène, -nodules tumoraux séparés dans deux lobes différents du même poumon.
N - Adénopathies	Nx	Envahissement locorégional inconnu.
	N0	Absence de métastase dans les ganglions lymphatiques régionaux.
	N1	Métastases ganglionnaires péri-bronchiques homolatérales et/ou hilaires homolatérales incluant une extension directe.
	N2	Métastases dans les ganglions médiastinaux homolatéraux ou dans les ganglions sous-carénaires
	N3	Métastases ganglionnaires médiastinales controlatérales ou hilaires controlatérales ou scaléniques, sus-claviculaires homo- ou controlatérales.
Métastases	M0	Pas de métastase à distance.
	M1	Existence de métastases :
	M1a	Nodules tumoraux séparés dans un lobe controlatéral, ou nodules pleuraux ou pleurésie maligne ou péricardite maligne
	M1b	1 seule métastase dans un seul site métastatique
	M1c	Plusieurs métastases dans un seul site ou plusieurs sites atteints

CLASSIFICATION PAR STADE

Carcinome occulte	Tx N0 M0	**Stade IIIA**	T1,2 N2, M0
Stade 0	Tis N0 M0		T3 N1 M0
Stade IA-1	T1a(mi) N0 M0		T4 N0,1 M0
	T1a N0 M0	**Stade IIIB**	T1,2 N3 M0
Stade IA-2	T1b N0 M0		T3,4 N2 M0
Stade IA-3	T1c N0 M0	**Stade IIIC**	T3,4 N 3 M0
Stade IB	T2a N0 M0	**Stade IV-A**	Tout M1a
Stade IIA	T2b N0 M0		Tout M1b
Stade IIB	T1,2 N1 M0	**Stade IV-B**	Tout M1c
	T3 N0 M0		

	N0	N1	N2	N3	M1a-b *Tout N*	M1c *Tout N*
T1a	IA-1	IIB	IIIA	IIIB	IV-A	IV-B
T1b	IA-2	IIB	IIIA	IIIB	IV-A	IV-B
T1c	IA-3	IIB	IIIA	IIIB	IV-A	IV-B
T2a	IB	IIB	IIIA	IIIB	IV-A	IV-B
T2b	IIA	IIB	IIIA	IIIB	IV-A	IV-B
T3	IIB	IIIA	IIIB	IIIC	IV-A	IV-B
T4	IIIA	IIIA	IIIB	IIIC	IV-A	IV-B

Appendix 4 Hospital Anxiety and Depression Scale (HAD)

1) نحس روحي على أعصابي و متوتر

A: 3 2 1 0

- ☐ دائما
- ☐ أغلب الأوقات
- ☐ مرّات
- ☐ لا أبدا

2) نستمتع بنفس الحوايج متاع قبل

D: 0 1 2 3

- ☐ نعم كيف العادة
- ☐ لا موش ياسر
- ☐ شوية شوية
- ☐ تقريبا بالكلّ

3) نحس بالخوف كأنه حاجة مرعبة باش تصير

A: 3 2 1 0

- ☐ نعم بالضبط
- ☐ نعم أما ما تماش خطر كبير
- ☐ شوية، أما موش متقلق من الحكاية
- ☐ لا أبدا

4) نضحك بسهولة ونشوف الناحية الإيجابية من الأشياء

D: 0 1 2 3

- ☐ نعم كيف العادة
- ☐ موش كيف العادة
- ☐ أقل ياسر من العادة
- ☐ لا أبدا

5) نخمم ونشغل روحي

A: 3 2 1 0

- ☐ دائما
- ☐ أغلب الأوقات
- ☐ مرات
- ☐ نادرا

6) نحس روحي مفرهد ومزاجي رائق

D: 0 1 2 3

- ☐ دائما
- ☐ أغلب الأوقات
- ☐ نادرا
- ☐ لا أبدا

7) نجم نقعد مرتاح ما نعمل شيء و نحس روحي مسترخي

A: 0 1 2 3

- ☐ نعم، مهما كانت الظروف
- ☐ نعم في أغلب الأوقات
- ☐ نادرا
- ☐ لا أبدا

8) نحس إني نمارس نشاطي بنسق بطيء على العادة

D: 3 2 1 0

- ☐ تقريبا دائما

- أغلى الأوقات
- مرّات
- لا أبدا

9) نحس بالخوف و ماعدتي معقودة (A: 0 1 2 3)

- لا أبدا
- مرّات
- ياسر
- دائما

10) ما عدتش نهتم بمظهري الخارجي (D: 3 2 1 0)

- لا أبدا
- موش كيف ما يلزم
- ممكن ساعات ما عدتش نهتم به
- نهتم كالعادة

11) نحس روحي ما نجمش نركح في بلاصة (A: 3 2 1 0)

- نعم بالضبط
- شوية
- شوية بالكل
- لا أبدا

12) نشيخ بالمسبق كيف نعرف روحي باش نعمل بعض الأشياء (D: 0 1 2 3)

- كيف العادة
- أقل شوية من العادة
- أقل ياسر من العادة
- لا أبدا

13) نحس بحالات رعب مفاجئ (A: 3 2 1 0)

- دائما
- ياسر مرّات
- موش ياسر ياسر
- لا أبدا

14) نجم نستمتع بقراءة كتاب باهي أو بالاستماع لبرنامج باهي في التلفزة والراديو (D: 0 1 2 3)

- دائما
- مرات
- نادرا
- نادر جدا

REFERENCES

1. **World health organization**. http://www.who.int/cancer/fr/.

2. **Krakowski.I, I.Boureau, F.Bugat, R.Chassignol, L.Colombat, P. Copel, Toussaint S et al** For a coordination of the supportive care for people affected by severe illnesses: proposal of organization in the public and private health care centres. 2004.Bull Cancer, 2004;91: 449-56.

3. **Michel-Nemitz J, Mazzocato C .** Treatment of cancer pain: a palliative approach. Swiss Medical Journal. 2005;25:1667-73.

4. **IASP Pain terms:** a list with definitions and notes on usage Recommended by International Association for study of Pain subcommittee on taxonomy. Pain. 1979;6:249-52.

5. **Bouhassira D, Attal N, Alchaar H, Boureau F, Brochet B, Bruxelle J,** et al. Comparison of pain syndromes associated with nervous or somatic lesions and development of a new neuropathic pain diagnostic questionnaire (DN4). Pain. 2005;114(1-2):29-36.

6. **Zigmond AS,** Snaith RP. The hospital anxiety and depression scale. Acta psychiatrica Scandinavica. 1983;67(6):361-70.

7. **World health organization.**
Cancer pain relief: with a guide to opioid availability. Geneva, second edition. 1996: 63.
http://www.who.int/iris/handle/10665/37896

8. **T.Delorme, C.Wood, A.Bataillard, E.Pichard, S.Dauchy, D.Orbach et** al. Recommendations for clinical practice: standards, options and recommendations for the assessment of pain in adults and children with cancer.National Federation of Pain Treatment Centres. 2003.

9. **Penet E, Javerliat M, Terrier G**
Pain assessment. In: Poulain P Douleur en oncologie Montrouge, John Libbey Eurotext. 2004:13- 24.

10. **Pichard-Léandri E,**
Assessment of pain in cancer patients . In: Brasseur L, Chauvin M, Guilbaud GPain: basic principles, pharmacology, acute pain, pain thérapeutiques Paris, Maloine. 1997:589-96.

11. **Caraceni A, Hanks G, Kaasa S, Bennett MI, Brunelli C, Cherny N, et al.** Use of opioid analgesics in the treatment of cancer pain: evidence-based recommendations from the EAPC. The Lancet Oncology. 2012;13(2):e58-68.

12. **Kitzis D.**
Pain management of cancer patients by general practitioners in Paris in 2012 [thesis]. Université Paris Est Créteil, Créteil Faculty of Medicine. 25 March 2012.

13. **Caraceni A.**
Evaluation and assessment of cancer pain and cancer pain treatment. Acta anaesthesiologica Scandinavica. 2001;45(9):1067-75.

14. **Conroy T, Mercier M, Bonneterre J, Luporsi E, Lefebvre JL, Lapeyre M, et al.** French version of FACT-G: validation and comparison with other cancer-specific instruments. European journal of cancer. 2004;40(15):2243-52.

15. **Kroenke K, Theobald D, Wu J, Loza JK, Carpenter JS, Tu W.**
The association of depression and pain with health-related quality of life, disability, and health care use in cancer patients.

Journal of pain and symptom management. 2010;40(3):327-41.

16. **Linton SJ, Bergbom S.**

Understanding the link between depression and pain. Scandinavian journal of pain. 2011;2(2):47-54.

17. **Fisch M.**

Treatment of depression in cancer. Journal of the National Cancer Institute Monographs. 2004(32):105-11.

18. **Fernandez E , Kerns RD**

Pain and affective disorders: looking beyond the "'chicken and egg'" conundrum. In: GiamberardinoM, Jensen TS, editors Pain comorbidities Seattle: IASP Press. 2012:279-96.

19. **Dropsy R, Marty M**.

Use of quality of life scales in chronic low back pain. Rev Rhum Mal Osteoartic. 1994;61:44S-8S.

20. **Agence nationale d'accréditation et d'évaluation en santé.**

Assessment and monitoring of chronic pain in adults in medicine ambulatoire. Paris: ANAES. 1999.

21. **Krakowsk I, Geoffrois L, Toussaint S**

Standards, options and recommendations 2002 on analgesic

drug treatments for cancer pain due to excess nociception in adults. Montrouge, John Libbey Eurotext. 2002:127.

22. **V. Piano , S. Verhagen, J. Burgers, H. Kress, R.-D. Treede, M. Lanteri- Minet,** Y. Engels, K. Vissers Diagnosis of pain neuropathic pain : comparison of recommendations for good practice in Europe. Proceedings of the SFETD congress, Lille, 21-24 November 2012.

23. **AFSSAPS.**
Good practice recommendations on intractable pain in advanced palliative care. Conditions of use, particularly outside the AMM, of certain drugs: permedullary, parenteral and topical local anaesthetics; fentanyl, sufentanil; ketamine; MEOPA; methadone; midazolam; permedullary and intracerebroventricular morphine; propofol. Paris: AFSSAPS. 2010.

24. **Beloeil H, Viel E, Navez ML, Fletcher D, Peronnet D**
Recommendations formalised of experts SFAR-SFETD. Techniques analgésiques locorégionales et douleur chronique: Guidelines for regional anaesthetic and analgesic techniques in the treatment of chronic pain syndromes Douleur Anal. 2013;26(2):110-20.

25. Lozeron P, Kubis N.

Management of neuropathic pain. The journal of internal medicine 2015;36:480-6.

26. Rostaing R, Guérin J.

Cancer pain: good clinical practice in management, management of strong opioids. The medical press. March 2014;Volume 43, No. 3.

27. RESO Nantes.

The general practitioner and cancer pain: testimony from a group of patients 53 GPs involved in pain management. Douleurs. 2007.

28. Liard F, Chassany O, Keddad K, Jolivet I.

Survey on pain management and training needs in general practice. Douelurs. Apr 2002;3(2):69-73.

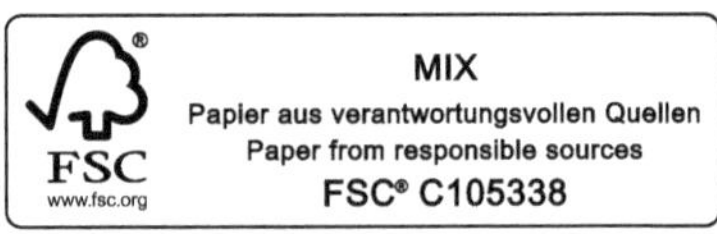

Printed by Books on Demand GmbH, Norderstedt / Germany